NATURAL STRESS BUSTERS

Options You May Not Know

By
Katherine Fletcher

INTRODUCTION

This book covers tips for reducing stress and enhancing your health. I have many suggestions for stress reduction as well as information about the main stressors in your body. Learn alternative ways to enhance your health through nutrition, aromatherapy, color, music, gemstone therapy and much more.

WHAT IS STRESS?

Stress is defined many different ways by many different people. Here are some of the definitions:

"Stress is an organism's total response to environmental demands or pressures." source: answer.com

"Stress is a normal psychological and physical reaction to the demands of life." source: revolutionhealth.com

"Stress is forces from the outside world impinging on the individual." source: medterms.com

MY DEFINITION OF STRESS

Stress is a natural part of life. It is the same as all our ups and downs in life. There are lessons to be learned and ways to continually improve your response to stress and the hard parts of life. Everyone has stress but the difference, in my opinion, is how you cope with the stress. How you deal with it, how you perceive, your attitude about it all play vital roles in handling your future stress. Stress can be a great motivator sometimes and can be a great teacher for us. There are many wonderful and joyous things in life like getting married, having a baby and moving that all are stressful but joyous.

Remember there is good stress too. There is always a lesson in it for us if we care enough to look deeper.

WHAT STRESS DOES IN THE BODY

Stress affects many organs and systems in the body. Adrenal glands are out of balance, the hypothalamus in the brain is affected, the hormones and neurotransmitters also incur some problems. Stress is about the "flight or fight response". Stress also affects the levels of serotonin, cortisol and DHEA and dopamine. It depletes many vitamins and minerals, especially B vitamins. Stress does weaken the immune system and makes it more difficult to fight infections and colds.

<u>Long term symptoms of stress can include:</u>

•heart disease

•sleep problems

•memory impairment

•depression

•digestive trouble

•obesity
•hormone problems

•high blood pressure

•skin problems

•tooth and gum disease

There are many factors that contribute to good health. Some of these include nutrition, less toxins in the body, exercise, a good diet and surrounding yourself with a group of happy and healthy friends. Emotions and attitude play a big role in optimal health.

We also know some of the things that stress the body the most. The blockers of healing so to speak. Many studies have done involving the five issues we will discuss first.

•Nutrition

•Toxins

•Food and environmental allergies

•Sugar and caffeine

•Emotions and Attitude

We will tackle these topics one at a time.

STRESS BUSTING TIPS

MY PERSONAL TIPS

One of my favorite tips is something I had to create for myself when I got too worried or stressed out.

Put your stress into categories.

1. Do I have any control over this situation?
   If you don't have control over it, let   it go. There is no use worrying about something you have no control over. If you're angry, get it   out and let it go. Acceptance of a situation is a huge part of controlling your stress level.

2. If you do have control over the situation then make a list of things you can do to fix the problem. If the problem seems too big, then divide into small steps.

3. My Worry Rule – give yourself 10 minutes to 1 hour daily just to worry if you want to. You are only allowed to worry during that time frame and then let it go. This takes practice but eliminates the worry that surrounds you all day.

   You've heard the saying to pick your battles – this applies to your stress also. You don't have to be stressed about everything...pick and choose which items are causing you the most stress. Then figure out how to resolve the issue or let it go. Ask yourself how much this issue is going to matter 10 years from now.

DEEP BREATHING TECHNIQUE

There are many good techniques and tips which I will provide you for reducing your stress. This is one of the techniques I use and also teach my clients.

Deep breathing is one of the quickest and easiest ways to relax. You can do it anywhere, anytime for any length of time. Scientists and doctors know that getting enough oxygen to all the organs can cause health problems. The amount of oxygen available to your cells is vital for optimum health. There is research that deep breathing helps with stress, PMS, depression, fertility and toxin elimination.

THE TECHNIQUE

•Lie flat on your back or sit in a chair with your back supported. You can also do this technique while working, walking, driving, etc.

•Place one hand on your abdomen and one hand on your chest.

•Inhale slowly and deeply (as is comfortable) through your nose into your abdomen. Hold it for 3 to 4 seconds. You should feel the hand on your abdomen move down and out, and only a slight movement of the hand on your chest. Exhale the breath slowly and completely.

•Repeat the above steps three times. Then inhale through your nose and exhale through your mouth, making a quiet whooshing sound (like the wind) as you blow out gently. Your tongue and jaw will be relaxed. Focus on the sound and feeling of breathing as you become more and more relaxed.

•Concentrate on your abdomen moving up and down, the air moving in and out of your lungs and the feelings of relaxation that deep breathing produces.

•You can try this breathing technique whenever you feel tense. Some people find that daily practice for 5 to 10 minutes at a time helps to master the technique.

One of the best programs I know and use to teach you how to breathe is called The Journey to the Wild Divine. This biofeedback program was developed by Deepak Chopra and several other doctors. It a fun computer game that is great for adults and kids. Much better than the video games your kids might be playing. It is beautiful, full animation and fantasy where each step teaches you a different kind of breath. Its affordable and great fun! Totally relaxing and healing for the body and mind.

POSITIVE AFFIRMATIONS

Affirmations or prayer are always helpful tools for reducing stress and enhancing health. An affirmation is a statement you make to yourself. In your mind or out loud. Repeat these over and over again and create your own affirmations based on your life. While meditating or visualizing is a good time to also use affirmations. They can help us to change many behaviors and thought patterns.

Health Affirmations:

I always contribute in healthy ways to my body.

I am living a long and healthy life.

I eat healthy, nutritious food every day.

I drink large amounts of water daily.

I have a healthy heart and a strong set of lungs.

God gave me a healthy body and I take care of it.

Peace Affirmations:

I am at peace with my choices in life.

I choose a peaceful and calm spirit.

I release my past and live with calm and serenity.

I am free to be me and express myself openly.

I have a peaceful and calming heart and soul.

My environment is a garden of peace.

The world is a peaceful, loving and enjoyable place to live.

Miscellaneous Life Affirmations:

I can accept whatever I feel today.

I listen with love and gratitude to my body's messages.

Love fills me and heals me and I open to connect with the people in my life.

I have the courage to look without fear at what needs to be changed in life.

Every experience is perfect for my growth process.

I release, relax and let go. I am safe here and now. I am safe in life.

I trust my inner wisdom. I listen to my own guidance.

I am confident and successful.

I encourage you to make your own list of affirmations based on the results YOU WANT in life. You can be specific as to your circumstance.

STRESS AND EMOTIONS

ATTITUDE is everything! It can be the biggest blocker to healing or the greatest healer of all. It depends on how you look at it, what your goals are and if you wear a positive attitude despite a sometimes tough road.

Visualization is a very important tool I use with my clients. The first step is to visualize your own perfect peaceful place. It can be a real place or a made up place, but it is yours alone. You can pick a beach with ocean waves, a green meadow with birds singing…anything you feel comfortable and relaxed in. Every time you get stressed out, close your eyes for a moment and go to this place in your mind. Take a few deep breathes by inhaling the goodness, peace and health (say this in your mind) and exhaling the negative energy, worry and fear.

You can use visualization for many things in life. Imagining your perfect job, what you might want your spouse or mate to be like and also to heal yourself. If you have an illness, injury or trauma visualize that in a form, shape or box. Visualize this and hit it with a hammer smashing it to bits (smashing the illness). You can also visualize the problem area or organ and see it healed and feeling great.

Emotions are also a big blocker of potential healing. We all have many traumas, difficult times and stress that takes its toll on our bodies and minds. The longer we hold onto to something, the more stress it causes our bodies. We have to learn to release emotion, NOT STUFF IT. Stuffing your emotions will make you sick and die younger. If you're not comfortable crying, find a quiet place where you can.

•Write the trauma in a journal and get it out.

•Write your fears down on a piece of paper and burn it, which releases it to the universe.

•Learn to forgive yourself and others. We all do the best we can with our circumstances.

•Figure out what lessons you learned from whatever trauma or hurt you're hanging onto. Once you understand the lessons it has served its purpose and it's time to let go.

THE VISUALIZATION TECHNIQUE

Imagery is a great method for reducing stress, especially when used in conjunction with deep breathing. The idea behind mental imagery is to create an enjoyable and relaxing environment in your mind. The more intensely you imagine the situation, the more relaxed you will be. Be involved in seeing, hearing, smelling - use all your senses when imagining.

When you imagine a pleasant scene you can see the changing levels of stress in your body through the biofeedback machine.

THE TECHNIQUE

•Imagine a scene, pace or event that you remember as peaceful. This could be a mountain stream, woods, fields, relaxing in a hot tub, etc. Anything that makes you feel peaceful and calm.

•You can also create mental pictures of stress flowing out of your Body or everyday concerns being locked in a chest.

•Breathe deeply and stay in this relaxing place for 15 minutes or so.

You can also use this technique for self-confidence.

VISUALIZATION

Visualizes uses the same technique as mental imagery, yet with some added applications. Athletes use visualization to see a victory in their minds before they play the game. Business professionals from all backgrounds use this technique to visualize the outcome of meetings or deals, personal success, financial success, etc. Visualization is a great tool for self-esteem, confidence and literally uses your thoughts to create your reality (quantum physics).

Visualize what you want - the outcome - and focus on all the positive things surrounding that image. You can create a bulletin board of your dreams or draw a picture so you can look at your dream.

MUSCLE RELAXATION TECHNIQUE

My next tip for reducing stress is the Progressive Muscle Relaxation technique. It takes a few times to get the hang of it, but it is great for stress and health. This is a useful technique for relaxing when your body is tense. Many times we don't realize how tense our muscles are.

THE TECHNIQUE

•Find a comfortable spot sitting or lying and do a few deep breaths.

•Start by forming a fist and clenching your hand as tight as you can for a few seconds. Then relax the hand by letting go.

•Repeat these steps with each muscle group. Tighten your arms, then relax; tighten your legs, then relax, etc. Also do your back, your facial muscles. Tighten, hold, then release and relax.

You can also use this technique when doing self-hypnosis for relaxation.

MEDITATION

Meditation refers to a state where your body and mind are consciously relaxed and focused. Practitioners of this art report increased awareness, focus, and concentration, as well as a more positive outlook in life.

Meditation is most commonly associated with monks, mystics and other spiritual disciplines. However, you don't have to be a monk or mystic to enjoy its benefits. And you don't even have to be in a special place to practice it. You could even try it in your own living room!

Although there are many different approaches to meditation, the fundamental principles remain the same. The most important among these principles is that of removing obstructive, negative, and wandering thoughts and fantasies, and calming the mind with a deep sense of focus. This clears the mind of debris and prepares it for a higher quality of activity.

The negative thoughts you have – those of noisy neighbors, bossy officemates, that parking ticket you got, and unwanted spam– are said to contribute to the 'polluting' of the mind, and shutting them out is allows for the 'cleansing' of the mind so that it may focus on deeper, more meaningful thoughts.

Some practitioners even shut out all sensory input – no sights, no sounds, and nothing to touch – and try to detach themselves from the commotion around them. You may now focus on a deep, profound thought if this is your goal. It may seem deafening at first, since we are all too accustomed to constantly hearing and seeing things, but as you continue this exercise you will find yourself becoming more aware of everything around you.

If you find the meditating positions you see on television threatening – those with impossibly arched backs, and painful-looking contortions – you need not worry. The principle here is to be in a comfortable position conducive to concentration. This may be while sitting cross-legged, standing, lying down, and even walking.

If the position allows you to relax and focus, then that would be a good starting point. While sitting or standing, the back should be straight, but not tense or tight. In other positions, the only no-no is slouching and falling asleep.

Loose, comfortable clothes help a lot in the process since tight fitting clothes have a tendency to choke you up and make you feel tense.

The place you perform meditation should have a soothing atmosphere. It may be in your living room, or bedroom, or any place that you feel comfortable in. You might want an exercise mat if you plan to take on the more challenging positions (if you feel more focused doing so, and if the contortionist in you is screaming for release). You may want to have the place arranged so that it is soothing to your senses.

Silence helps most people relax and meditate, so you may want a quiet, isolated area far from the ringing of the phone or the humming of the washing machine. Pleasing scents also help in that regard, so stocking up on aromatic candles isn't such a bad idea either.

The monks you see on television making those monotonous sounds are actually performing their mantra. This, in simple terms, is a short creed, a simple sound which, for these practitioners, holds a mystic value.

You do not need to perform such; however, it would pay to note that focusing on repeated actions such as breathing, and humming help the practitioner enter a higher state of consciousness.

The principle here is focus. You could also try focusing on a certain object or thought, or even, while keeping your eyes open, focus on a single sight.

One sample routine would be to – while in a meditative state – silently name every part of your body and focusing your consciousness on that part. While doing this you should be aware of any tension on any part of your body. Mentally visualize releasing this tension. It works wonders.

In all, meditation is a relatively risk-free practice and its benefits are well worth the effort (or non-effort – remember we're relaxing).

Studies have shown that meditation does bring about beneficial physiologic effects to the body. And there has been a growing consensus in the medical community to further study the effects of such. So in the near future, who knows, that mystical, esoteric thing we call meditation might become a science itself!

MUSIC THERAPY

Music has been known to effect the body and mind in many ways. It is because each musical note has its own frequency which in turn causes our brain to react in certain ways.

There have been numerous studies done on the effects of music on the mind and body. The results are amazing.

Soft music will calm and soothe you and is great for stress. Singing out loud will also help you feel better.

Rock and Roll music will give you energy and motivation.

Specific music such as Beethoven and Bach does wonders for your brain and body.

MASSAGE THERAPY

Massage therapy is the ultimate relaxation tool. It helps relax the body and mind. In addition to helping your sore muscles massage is known to increase your health and relax the mind. Massage tends to get some toxins out of your body which is beneficial for your overall health.

I am a Massage Therapist and see daily the stress relief my clients get.

REIKI ENERGY WORK

Reiki is an energy treatment for the mind and body. It is non-invasive and usually hands on. It is the process of bringing healing energy into your body and ensuring that body's energy is in balance. Certain organs and/or emotional issues often show up as blocked energy in the body.
Clearing these energy blockages will allow your body to function better.

My clients love Reiki. It is super relaxing and often helps certain issues with the body.

GET ORGANIZED

One of the most important steps to making your life simple is to get organized. You would be amazed at the difference it makes in your life when you get rid of the excess clutter and get yourself organized.

How to organize paperwork

If you don't already have a filing cabinet or a filing box then get one. This is an easy way to store important files. You should have files for your house, car, utility, taxes, cable payments as well as any credit cards. Each of your accounts should have a separate file. You should also keep a file for important documents. Make a copy of your driver's license, SS card, birth certificate, passport information and the front and back of your credit cards. In case your wallet is stolen or lost you can access that information easily.

Organize garage & household

Think about the options of plastic storage containers for holiday stuff and extra items.

Storage containers come in a variety of sizes and can be found at many local stores. Plain wooden boards can be used to make shelving in the garage for tools and other items. I often use inexpensive baskets and old milk crates to store and organize my stuff. You can also buy pre-fabricated shelving and paint it. Spend some time going through your house and garage. Ask yourself what do you really use, want and need?

Part of the process of getting rid of the clutter is to get rid of stuff that no longer serves you. Make a list of what you have, what to sell, what to give away and what to keep.

While cleaning out your garage, attic or basement you can make separate piles or boxes for the items you are selling, donating and keeping.

A great way to sell your extra stuff is to list it on free local classified ads or craigslist. Another option is to take the items to a local flea market or auction house to sell. The donation pile should be taken to Goodwill or your local Salvation Army store and they will give you a tax deduction receipt. Next, think about the items you are keeping and how you want to use them in your house.

OTHER EASY STRESS REDUCING TIPS

- Take a hot bath with a little lavender oil for relaxation

- Read a great book

- Take a Nap

- Sunshine

- Walks in the woods or parks

- Get a massage

- Pamper yourself

- Laugh Every day

- Be grateful and thank people

I want to let you know that YouTube has many great videos for relaxation, meditation, color therapy and more. Just watching these specialty videos will help your stress and health.

PAMPER YOURSELF WITH THIS IDEA

SIMPLE BEAUTY can be achieved in many natural ways. Using natural soap and lotion help cut down on the toxins in your body. Make your skin happy with natural soap, shampoo and these great natural face masks.

HERBAL FACE MASKS

Instead of spending a fortune on expensive face creams and peel masks, why not do it yourself? Save money and make life simple. Here are some great herbal face masks you can make!

WHOLE EGG PACK

- Beat up a whole egg until frothy.
- Apply to clean, dry face.
- Let it dry and rinse it off.

OATMEAL OR CORNMEAL PACK

- Mix a little oatmeal with water or egg white and apply to face.
- Scrub areas around nose and chin
- Let dry 15 minutes
- Rinse with tepid water, rose water or orange water.

TOMATO PACK

- Slice one large tomato into thick slices

- Let juice and seeds drain off
- Mash tomato slices and apply to face
- Lay hot washcloth over face for 15 minutes
- Rinse off with tepid water

CUCUMBER FACE PACK

- Cut a cucumber into thin long strips
- Apply strips to face
- Cover with hot washcloth
- Keep washcloth on until cold
- Rinse with cucumber water or witch-hazel extract

YOGURT FACIAL PACK

- Mix yogurt with a dash of lemon juice.
- Apply to face
- Let stand for 10 to 20 minutes
- Rinse and add dash of cucumber water, rose water or elder flower water

HONEY AND EGG PACK

- Beat an egg white with a few grams of alum camphor or menthol.
- Cover face with egg white and let it dry
- Keep on for 15 to 20 minutes
- Rinse thoroughly and dry
- Apply organic honey to the face
- Keep on for 5 minutes
- Rinse with orange flower water or elder flower water

ALTERNATIVE THERAPIES

STRESS AND COLOR THERAPY

Color Therapy is a complementary therapy for which there is evidence dating back thousands of years to the ancient cultures of Egypt, China and India. Color is simply light of varying wavelengths, thus each color has its own particular wavelength and energy. You can get colored light bulbs, use clothing, flowers to expose yourself to color. If you need energy and stimulation wear a red shirt that day. Sometimes I'll buy the flowers of the colors I want around my house.

The Color **RED** is great for circulation, kidneys, heart, Muscles, chronic illness and bone strengthening.

The Color **ORANGE** relates to joy and happiness, creativity and generosity. It is a great color for depression and a known relaxer

The color **YELLOW** is great for learning and mental activity. It enhances focus and concentration, confidence and empowerment. This color is great for combating fears, aids digestion and helps the gall bladder, liver and nervous system.

The color **GREEN** is calming, soothing and sedative. It also involves money/prosperity, new beginnings and healing. Green is great for the liver, anti-inflammatory and promotes eye health and strong bones.

The color **TURQUOISE** is great for self-respect and unconditional love. It is good for the skin, mental relaxation and regulates the large intestine systems.

The color **BLUE** is calming and brings deep inner peace. It stimulates higher mental activities and provides insight and wisdom. Blue is a great anti-bacterial and helps headaches and insomnia.

The color **VIOLET** is great for meditation and inspiration. It provides an inner emotional release and stimulates dreams. Violet is great for menopause, spleen and solar plexus.

The color **White or Clear** actually contains all colors. White helps everything on all levels including spiritual/physical/mental. It is about innocence, purity and radiance.

AROMATHERAPY

Aromatherapy is a great tool for stress relief. The sense of smell is very important for health and stress reduction. You can buy scented candles, like lavender which are relaxing. Scents are everywhere. One of the ways to get smells is through essential oils.

Essential oils have been used for thousands of years. There is a risk to using them so you must be careful and learn more about it. The essential oils are highly concentrated and MUST BE MIXED WITH CARRIER OILS before using. My recommendation is to buy the oil combinations already mixed and ready to use.

CARRIER OILS

Carrier oils are the base oil you use to start with and the a few drops of the flower essences are added to it. Flower essences are very concentrated therefore must be added sparingly to a carrier oil. Some examples of carrier oils are grape seed, sunflower, sweet almond, flaxseed and olive oil. Carrier oils have a shelf life of about one year and should be kept in the refrigerator.

WAYS TO USE IT

On the skin = with massage therapy, mixed with carrier oil on the skin. Sometimes you have to mix with other oils, some you can use directly on the skin. Some of them have high heat effect.

SMELL IT

Use a diffuser to disperse the smell in the air. Only run for a limited time, no more than 2 hours because of medicinal effects. You can steam eucalyptus in a pan of boiling water to inhale when you have a cold.

LEMON OIL

Lemon oil is also cold pressed like cedar oil. Lemon oil is used for athlete's foot, colds, flu, oily skin and spots. It is also used for varicose veins and warts. It is anti-bacterial, anti-viral and anti-inflammatory. It's great for hypertension. Do not use it if the area of skin application will be exposed to sunlight for 24 hours. It is a phototoxic oil. It may cause skin irritation with some people. All citrus oils are phototoxic.

LAVENDER OIL

Lavender oil is steam distilled from the lavender flower. It has a fresh, sweet floral smell. Lavender oil has anti-inflammatory properties. It is used for a variety of conditions including skin, headaches, hypertension and anxiety. It has a very calming effect. Lavender is also used for allergies, bruises, burns, cuts, earaches and insect bites. In relation to massage lavender oil is great for scars, sores, sprains, strains and muscle aches.

EUCALYPTUS

Eucalyptus has antibacterial, antiviral and anti-rheumatic properties. It is used for asthma, colds and congestion. Eucalyptus is also used for migraines, headaches, pain relief and for wounds and burns. One of the ways to use

Eucalyptus is to steam it in a pot of boiling water and inhale it deeply.

ROSEMARY

Rosemary oil comes from steam distillation and has a clear color. It is an analgesic and anti-inflammatory. It is used for aching muscles, arthritis, exhaustion, gout, hair and skin, bronchitis and colds. Rosemary is also known to help circulation, headaches and muscle cramping. It is a neuro-toxin and should never be used with pregnant women, epilepsy or fever. It should not be taken internally.

CLARY SAGE

Clary sage has anti-bacterial and antispasmodic properties. It is used for calming and depression, headaches, menstrual cramps and PMS as well as muscle stress. It is used medicinally for asthma, coughs, sore throats and exhaustion. It is also helpful for labor pains and stress. This oil has a sedative effect and should not be used while driving or drinking alcohol.

SANDLEWOOD

Sandalwood is steam distilled and is used for bronchitis, skin and stretch marks. In addition, it is helpful for depression and stress. Sandalwood is also used for insomnia and meditation and calming. It also has anti-bacterial properties.

** There are many different scents available with aromatherapy.   These are just a few of the most common ones.

GEMSTONE THERAPY

Crystal and gem therapy is the use of semiprecious and precious stones to enhance mental, spiritual, and physical healing. It is based on the belief that certain crystals and gems possess a powerful vibrational frequency energy that can positively affect imbalances in human energy fields and thus promote health and well-being. Some stones effect emotional states, while others affect certain organs. It all

Gemstone Therapy has nevertheless been used for centuries by astrologers, diviners, priests, Buddhist monks, and others. Today the stones are employed not only by crystal and gemstone therapists, but also by some reflexologists, aroma therapists, kinesiologists, spiritual healers, and other alternative practitioners.

There more than 200 other stones used in crystal and gem therapy as well.

Amazonite - Improves self-worth

Amber - Lift heaviness. Amber is great at lifting the heaviness of burdens allowing happiness to come through.

Amethyst: - Spiritual Upliftment. This is also the present carrier of the purple color ray. Also helpful with stomach issues.

Aquamarine – This is a great stone for those experiencing great loss and grief.

Aventurine – Circulation and congestion.

Green Aventurine – is used for physical healing

Citrine – Upliftment and to help align the spine

Coral - Emotional Foundation. Coral protects and strengthens one's emotional foundation.

Diamond - Increase personal clarity

Emerald - Physical and emotional healing. This is the strongest physical healing gemstone.

Green Fluorite - Hormone Balance. This stone is helpful with hormonal changes such as PMS and menopause.

Jade - Relaxation.

Malachite - Bring harmony into one's life.

Moss Agate - Get in touch with nature.

Mother of Pearl – Protection

Black Obsidian - Grounding stone

Black Onyx - Helps one to change bad habits.

Opal – allows us to see all the possibilities in a given situation.

Rose Quartz – is great for Emotional balance

Rhodonite - Emotional support.

Ruby –involves Love and opening the heart

Sapphire - Mental clarity.

Sunstone – Enhances dreams and contemplations

Quart – rose quart, clear and Smokey quartz are all great for emotional stability.

Discover the properties of unknown stones for yourself. Find out what is true for you. Keep your stone with you as much as possible for a week. Place it next to your bedside when you sleep at night; wear it or put it on your desk during the day.

OTHER STRESS FACTORS

Nutrition, Toxins, Allergies & More

NUTRITION

You can conquer lots of stress by feeding yourself the right foods and getting the proper amount of vitamins and minerals your body needs.   It is important to know your vitamins and which foods contain certain vitamins. You can focus on your specific health issues by focusing in on the vitamins/minerals you need the most.

VITAMIN CHART

CHART OF VITAMINS AND FUNCTION

VITAMIN A - acne, skin, eyes, respiratory, cancer prevention

B1 Thiamine -nerve problems, Beriberi, heart muscle, edema, energy

B2 Riboflavin - inflammation of skin, eyes, and nerves, depression, dementia

B3 Niacin -Pellagra, scaly dermatitis white, nerve disease, dementia, wild

B4 Niacin amide - digestion, dementia, skin irritation, diarrhea, irritable bowel

B5 Pantothenic acid - coordination, adrenal function, energy, unfocused thought

B6 Pyridoxine - convulsions anemia, irritability, cannot remember dreams

B7 Folic acid - digestive disease, anemia, energy, hormone function, moody

B8 Coenzyme A - energy management, adrenal thyroid and pituitary function

B9 PABA - skin, energy, loss of motor neuron function, depression

B10 Biotin Vitamin H - mental and muscle problems, chronic fatigue

B11 Inositol - master molecule of carbon regulation and liver function

B12 Dibencozide - pernicious anemia, white blood cell function, immunity

B13 Choline - digestion, stomach function, gall bladder depression

B14 Betaine - nerves of digestion and liver depression

B15 Panmagic acid - oxygenation disease, itching, liver function, lungs

B16 Oxythiamine - oxygenation energy regulation

B17 Laetrile - degeneration regulation of oxygenation

B18 FAD - oxygenation, energy regulation eye function)

B19 Flavin Mononucleotide - immunity, oxygenation, energy

B20 Carnitine - oxygenation, heart muscle, energy regulation in muscles

VITAMIN C - cancer prevention, bones, viral and bacterial infections, gums, allergy, cholesterol, gums

VITAMIN D - bone and teeth, nerve and muscle formation, bowel, breast and cancer prevention

VITAMIN E - blood clots, scar formation, nerves and brain, wound healing, cancer prevention

VITAMIN K - blood clotting, reduces bleeding

VITAMIN P - bruising and bleeding, stabilizes vitamin C, prevents cataract formation

OTHERS

OMEGA 3 - heart disease, triglyceride, arthritis,

VITAMIN & MINERAL FOOD SOURCES

Our soil is mostly depleted of minerals, but if you grow your own or buy organic you will get some vitamins and minerals. Check the country of origin labels now required to be on fruits, veggies, meat and seafood. Don't get seafood from China. Don't get fruits from Chile. They use too many pesticides and insecticides to make it safe for eating.

VITAMIN / MINERAL FOOD SOURCE

Protein - Chicken, soybeans, fish, ham, beef, cottage cheese

Carbohydrates - Whole grains, honey, syrup, fruits, veggies

Vitamin A - Liver, dark green leafy veggies, cantaloupe, sweet Potato, carrots, spinach, chard, tomato, eggs

Vitamin B1 - Brewer's yeast, dry soybeans, ham, wheat germ, sunflower seeds, fortified cereals, Brazil nuts, oatmeal

Vitamin B2 - Liver, organic meat, mushrooms, skim milk, eggs, beef, cottage cheese, chicken, spinach, ham, fortified cereals

Vitamin B3 - Salmon, tuna, chicken, halibut, liver, peanuts, all brain mushrooms, other fish, brewer's yeast

Vitamin B4 - Soybeans, fresh salmon, canned salmon, molasses, Liver, wheat bran, beef, cod, sunflower seeds

Vitamin B5 - Liver, organic meats, eggs, soybeans, broccoli, peanuts, mushrooms, beef, haddock, brewer's yeast

Vitamin B10 - egg yolks, liver, unpolished rice, brewer's yeast, whole grains, sardines, legumes

Vitamin B11 - whole grains, citrus fruits, brewer's yeast, molasses, meat, milk, nuts, veggies

Vitamin B12 -liver, beef kidney, oysters, salmon, fresh sole, chicken, ham, pork

Vitamin C - Broccoli, green pepper, hot peppers, Brussels sprouts, cantaloupe, dark green leafy veggies, citrus fruit or juice, strawberries, cabbage, watermelon

Vitamin D - Salmon, sardines, herring, milk, egg yolks, sunshine, organic meats

Vitamin E - soybean oil, corn or cottonseed oil, wheat germ, peanuts, margarine, mayonnaise, broiled salmon steak

Vitamin F - vegetable oils, butter, sunflower seeds

Vitamin K - Green leafy veggies, egg yolks, safflower oil, blackstrap molasses, cauliflower, soybeans

Vitamin P - citrus fruits, other fruits, black currants, buckwheat

Vitamin T - sesame seeds, raw sesame butter, egg yokes

Vitamin U - raw cabbage juice, fresh cabbage, homemade Sauerkraut

SOME OF THE MINERALS

Choline - Egg yolks, organic means, wheat germ, soybeans, fish, and legumes

Calcium - Milk, broccoli, dark green leafy veggies, cheese, molasses, legumes, almonds, cottage cheese, Brazil nuts

Potassium - Soybeans, cantaloupe, sweet potato, avocado, raisins, banana, halibut, sole, baked beans, molasses, ham, mushrooms, beef, and white potatoes.

Magnesium - Soybeans, wheat germ, cashews, almonds, Brazil nuts, baked beans, peanuts, molasses, dark green leafy veggies

Sodium - Seafood, table salt, sea salt, baking powder, baking soda, celery, milk products, kelp

Phosphorus - Tuna, sweetbreads, wheat germ, soybeans, fried beef liver, Brazil nuts, beef

Copper - Organic meats, seafood, nuts, legumes, molasses, raisins, bone meal

Zinc - Beef, oatmeal, dark chicken, fish, beef liver, dried beans, bran, tuna

Iron - Prune juice, liver, beef, soybeans, baked beans, ham, organic meats, chicken, spinach, eggs

Manganese - Whole grains, green leafy veggies, legumes, nuts, pineapples, egg yokes

Cobalt - Organic meals, oysters, clams, poultry, milk, green leafy veggies, fruits

Chromium - Corn oil, clams, whole grain cereals, brewer's yeast

Selenium - Tuna, herring, brewer's yeast, wheat germ and bran, broccoli, whole grains

Chlorine - table salt, seafood, meats, ripe olives, rye flour

Sulfur - Fish, eggs, meats, cabbage, Brussels sprouts

Fluoride - tea, seafood, water, bone meal

Molybdenum - Legumes, whole grain cereals, milk, liver, dark green veggies

Vanadium - Fish

Iodine - Iodized salt, ocean fish

Tryptopan - soy protein, chicken, soybeans, fish, eggs, vegetable patty, cottage cheese, milk, mixed nuts, baked beans

Leucine - Beef, chicken, soy protein, fish, soybeans, ham, cottage cheese, liver, eggs, baked beans

Lysine - Chicken, beef, fish, ham, soy protein, soybeans, cottage cheese, baked beans, eggs, goat milk, peanuts, oatmeal, and brewer's yeast

Threonine - beef, chicken, fish, ham, soy protein, soybeans, liver, eggs, cottage cheese, goat milk, baked beans, veggie patty.

Valine - beef, chicken, fish, soy protein, soybeans, ham, eggs, liver, veggie patty, cottage cheese, baked beans, milk

Methionine - chicken, beef, fish, ham, eggs, cottage cheese, liver, soybeans, soy protein, veggie patty, sardines, milk, yogurt

VITAMIN ROBBERS
What depletes and snatches our vitamins?

Everyone has heard of vitamins all over the world, but few of us think in terms of anti-vitamins or substances that rob our bodies of these essential nutrients. Chemicals in food, water, polluted air, common medicines, drugs, laxatives, refined sugar and flour, alcohol, coffee and caffeinated beverages, chocolates, the pill, tobacco and stress are all good examples of these culprits.

- Air Pollution

- Alcohol

- Stress

- Sugar

- Antacids

- Antibiotics

- Aspirin

- Chlorine

- Coffee (Caffeine)

- Fish and shell fish (raw)

- Fluorides

- Menustration

- Nitrates

- Oral Contraceptives

- Tobacco

- Penicillin

MINERALS AND STRESS

Minerals are vitally necessary for the body to function. Doctors know that STRESS depletes the body of certain minerals. It especially affects the adrenal glands so pay attention to which minerals support the adrenals.

Let's first learn about what each mineral's function is in the body.

MINERAL CHART

Calcium - weak bones, nerves, adrenals

Potassium - fatigue, nerves, energy, heart

Sodium - depression, nerves, fatigue, digestion

Chlorine - acid/alkaline balance, stomach acid, nerves

Magnesium - adrenal regulation, oxygen energy

Iron - anemia, fatigue, oxygen

Sulphur - detox, energy, emotions, unfocused

Manganese - nerve and muscle disease

Chromium - sugar regulation, muscle

Zinc - immunity, oxygen, metabolic disease

Selenium - detox, nerves, energy, skin

Iodine - thyroid function, energy, metabolism

Phosphorous - cellular function, energy, thought

Boron - nerve regulation dementia depression

Molybedum - thyroid function, lactation, fatigue

Silicon - bone, skin, nerves

Cobalt - anemia, immunity

Lithium - nerves, thought, energy, hypothalamus

Germanium - nerves, oxygenation, skin, energy

Arsenic - energy, nerves

Antimony - skin, detox, bowel function

Tin - nerves, muscles

Carbon - energy, life regulation

Vanadium - liver function heart muscle

Aluminum - nerves, thought regulation

Copper - nerves, energy, detox

Nickel - liver function heart muscle

Gold - detox, thought regulation

Silver - immunity, energy, detox

Amino Acids also play an important role in many functions of the body. It is important to have all the necessary vitamins, minerals, aminos and fatty acids that the body needs.

AMINO ACIDS

Phenylalanine - pain control, nerves

Alanine - kidney and nerves

Cysteine - kidney utilization

Leucine - mood control, emotions

Isoleucine - emotional control, nerves

Serine - carbohydrate energy conversion

Tryptophan - serotonin and relaxation

Histidine - antiinflamation, antiallergy

Methionine - liver and oxygenation

Lysine - anti herpes lesion, nerves

Threonine - hormonal and energy production

Tyrosine - thyroid and adrenal function

Valine - for regulation of blood cells

Glutamine - supplies energy to brain

Proline - sulphur disorders

Arginine - nerves and skin

Glutamine Acid - supplies energy to brain

Aspartic Acid - NutraSweet, nerve destruction

Adenosine - circulation, energy

Uracil - for RNA function

Adenine - for DNA RNA function

Guanine - for DNA RNA function

Cytosine - for DNA RNA function

Thymine - for DNA RNA function

Tryptophan - mood control, energy, healing, sleep

Taurine - energy

Citruline - thinking

GABA - thought control

STRESS AND ALLERGIES

One of the biggest sources of stress in the body are allergies. Allergic reactions can result from foods, insect stings, and reactions to medications like aspiring and antibiotics such as penicillin. There are also pollen, flower and chemical allergies. An allergy is defined as a disorder of the immune system. Allergic reactions occur to environmental substances known as allergens.

FOOD ALLERGIES

Food allergies are very important and can cause lots of physical and mental problems. Wheat allergies and dairy are very common and can really create stress in the body. In fact many studies show that Attention Deficit Disorder, brain fog and behavioral problems are common in children with wheat and dairy allergies. Symptoms of food allergy include abdominal pain, bloating, vomiting, diarrhea, itchy skin and more. Food allergies rarely cause respiratory (asthmatic) reactions, or rhinitis.

Milk allergy is the most common food allergy in early childhood. It affects somewhere between 2% and 3% of infants in developed countries, but approximately 85-90% of affected children lose clinical reactivity to milk once they surpass 3 years of age. Between 13% and 20% of children allergic to milk are also allergic to beef. Soy milk is a good option to cow's milk.

POLLEN / SEASONAL ALLERGIES

Many allergens such as dust or pollen are airborne particles. In these cases, symptoms arise in areas in contact with air, such as eyes, nose and lungs. For instance, allergic rhinitis, also known as hay fever, causes irritation of the nose, sneezing, and itching and redness of the eyes. Inhaled allergens can also lead to asthmatic symptoms, caused by narrowing of the airways and increased production of mucus in the lungs, shortness of breath), coughing and wheezing.

CHEMICALS AND OTHER ALLERGENS

Substances that come into contact with the skin, such as latex, are also common causes of allergic reactions, known as contact dermatitis or eczema. Skin allergies frequently cause rashes, or swelling and inflammation within the skin. Other frequent dermatitis allergies relate to scented lotion and the chemicals contained in lotion and soap. Some people are allergic to certain fragrances and odors such as perfumes. Many common environmental allergies are caused by pollution, such as carbon monoxide and gas fumes.

SOLUTIONS

You can go to an allergist and get tested for a variety of foods to determine what you allergic too. Or you can listen to your body and do some experimenting. Pay attention to how you feel after consuming wheat or dairy. Sluggish, tired, brain fog, digestive problems? Then try eliminating dairy or wheat from your diet for two weeks. See how you feel now. You can certainly learn to reduce the amount of wheat and dairy you consume if this is an allergy or sensitivity for you. You can also reduce your exposure to chemical and environmental pollution, use scent and chemical free soap and lotion for your skin and dust your house more frequently. Mold and house dust is a common allergen for most people.

STRESS AND PARASITES

PARASITES AND WORMS

I know we don't like to think about it, but we all have parasites and worms. Many of us don't realize how much harm to the body these little critters can cause. Parasites and worms are also one of the major causes of stress and illness in the body. A parasite is an organism that lives off another organism. In this case, they live off our cells, energy, nutrition and more.

Where Do We Get Parasites?

Parasites come from our food, water, pets, gardens and other sources. They are found worldwide. Poor sanitation doesn't help but we still can acquire worms through every day activities. Walking barefoot in the garden, contact with pets, meats, certain fruits and veggies (depending on the soil). Our water supply can also be infected, also swimming in lakes and oceans. Most parasites and worms are microscopic so we don't visually see them. Worms can release as many as 200,000 eggs per day. Think about that for a minute.

Once they get in our body they can settle into our organs, sap our nutrition. The intestinal tract is the most common area for worms and parasites to settle. Parasites reproduce around the full moon so this is when we feel the effect the most. Our bodies may actually play host to over 100 different types of parasites.

Types of Parasites / Worms

Roundworms

It is estimated that 25% of the world's population has roundworms. They get infections from consuming worm eggs found on fruits and veggies in contaminated soil.

Some of the symptoms of roundworms are intestinal gas, weight gain around full moon, digestive problems, fatigue, anemia, teeth grinding and blood sugar imbalances.

Tapeworms

There are lots of different types of tapeworms and they can grow to be very large in the body. The usually source of tapeworms is pork, beef and also our pets. When they get in our intestines, the absorb all of our nutrients and the give off dangerous waste.

Some of the symptoms of tapeworms are thyroid and intestinal imbalances, blood sugar imbalances, jaundice, bloating, gas and a possible fluid buildup during the full moon.

Flukes

These are very small parasites that attach themselves to our organs. Some of these organs include the lungs, heart, intestines, brain, bladder, liver and blood vessels which can cause inflammation and damage. The eggs are tiny with protruding spines that cause damage as they move through the body. The main source of flukes is raw or under cooked fish or crab, infected veggies like water chestnuts or drinking and wading through infected water.

Single Cell parasites

These are also called Protozoans and these microscopic critters cause more harm than any other kind of parasite. Our immune systems usually naturally take care of these parasites, but if your body and immune system is weak, you have a better chance of having them. They are very resistant to dryness, chemicals and temperature which are everywhere in our society. Protozoans are found in the intestines, muscle tissue, digestive tract and lungs. They release toxins and tissue destroying enzymes. Infections caused by Protozoans are associated with arthritis, asthma, Hodgkin's lymphoma, M.S., ovarian cysts, dermatitis, muscle diseases and more.

GETTING RID OF THESE NASTY PARASITES

Herbal cleanses are great for getting rid of worms and parasites. I also recommend limiting or eliminating the amount of pork from your diet. This seems to be a huge source from our foods. Herbal cleanses should be started a week before the full moon, since parasites reproduce at the full moon. It is important to stay on a 4 to 5 week cleanse to ensure you get the next full moon to get rid of the remaining eggs.

Some suggestions:

* eating raw pumpkin seeds to keep parasites away

* Garlic, thyme, cayenne also help with parasites.

* Milk Thistle and cloves are also great for parasites and restoring the digestive tract.

* avoid sugar and alcohol and potato chips which parasites love and thrive on.

* Pomegranates, cranberry juice, apple cider vinegar are good foods to control parasites

STRESS AND TOXINS

Toxins are a huge problem stressing out the body. They come from many sources. Toxins cause our vitamins and minerals to be depleted and cause many physical problems. Here are some of the sources of toxins are how you are getting exposed.

Lead – in makeup, lipstick, lead toys from China, old paint, in water sometimes,

Mercury – from tuna, oysters sometimes, dental fillings

Aluminum – from deodorant, from cookware,

Environmental Pollution – from factories, cars and city pollution

Insecticides and Pesticides – City parks, ball fields, and golf courses are the worst culprits of exposure. Don't spray chemicals on your own lawns. There are natural green based insecticides available in every city now.

Drinking Water – get a filter to get out some of the lead and other particles.

Chlorine – from swimming pools and your water. Get a chlorine filter for your shower so it won't absorb into the skin. In addition, with the steam of the shower you also end up inhaling the chlorine into the lungs.

Beauty Shop Toxins – Use natural soap, shampoo, conditioners, gel, hair spray and makeup if possible. There are numerous chemicals in the regular hair care products that end up absorbing partially into your brain. This is a big source of brain toxins and you can avoid it. IN a recent study of a general population who got their blood tested, many had very high levels of a certain chemical found in soap, shampoo, lotions. Scientists were shocked to see levels so high. There are organic soaps, deodorants and food you can buy to limit your exposure to toxins.

REMEMBER TOXINS ARE ABSORBED THROUGH THE SKIN and NOSE

 What you touch and smell are important. Heavy metals - especially aluminum have been linked to Alzheimer's disease. * Household maintenance Glue, stain, paint, caulking Mold and mildew in the homes

* Cleaning Products all cleaning products have chemicals and toxins - use latex gloves Avoid microwave use Avoid plastic food containers, plastic wrap and plastic water bottles

* Food - many foods have toxins and chemicals in them. The worst of foods sprayed are strawberries, bell peppers, spinach, peaches, green beans, cucumbers, apples, celery.

* Water Try drinking clean filtered water, not tap water don't drink out of plastic water bottles

You can do something about your toxins. Let your feet sweat which gets out lots of toxins through the pores of your feet. Go without anti-perspirant when you can and let yourself sweat.

Avoid or limit your time on golf courses, ball fields, city parks which are all sprayed heavily with pesticides and insecticides.

Get a chlorine filter for your shower to help reduce the amount of chlorine your skin and lungs are absorbing.

SUGAR IS A HUGE PROBLEM

If you've listened to the news reports lately you'll know there is a war on sugar.   White processed sugar is terrible for us in many ways.   There are many studies on the internet and in health magazines you can read to learn more.

I recommend to get Sugar in the Raw or Stevia for a sugar substitute. Avoid the sodas and avoid the additive Aspartame which is now being used as a sugar substitute. Check the labels, even on your chewing gum and breath mints to ensure there is no aspartame.

About the Author

Katherine Fletcher is a freelance writer and Massage Therapist. She lives in the mountains of NC.

OTHER BOOKS
BY KATHERINE FLETCHER

Genealogy Books

The Rice Family History – From Ireland to VA, NC and TN

The Turnage Family History – from Essex, England to VA, NC, SC and West Tennessee

The Trent Family History –England to VA to East TN

England/McKinney & Little Family History – West Tennessee

Regular Books

Real Treasure Hunting for Beginners

Make Life Simple

Scenes From the West

Aunt Irene's Secret Southern Recipes

Children's books

What Happens When We Die?

Why Do People Eat? A Children's Lesson in Nutrition

All of these books can be ordered through Amazon.com and are available as a Kindle download.